To
Dave & Peggy,

Thank you for your
commitment to marria
May the Lord richly bl

Keeping Covenant,
Oscar & Crystal Jones

MW00978030

When The Vow
Breaks

Discover how to restore hope and
healing in your marriage

by

Oscar & Crystal Jones

When The Vow
Breaks

Discover how to restore hope and
healing in your marriage

by

Oscar & Crystal Jones

Destiny House Publishing
Detroit, Michigan

When The Vow Breaks

Published by Destiny House Publishing, LLC
Copyright © 2003 Oscar and Crystal Jones
International Standard Book Number: 145054214X

Unless otherwise stated, all scripture quotations are from The Holy Bible, New King James Version. Scripture references that do not have the Bible version noted are the author's paraphrase.

Original printing August 2003
Cover design. Editing and Publication Layout:
Destiny House Publishing, LLC. ALL RIGHTS RESERVED

All rights reserved

All rights reserved under International Copyright law. No part of this book may be reproduced or transmitted in any form or by any means: electronic, mechanical, including photocopying and recording, or by any information storage and retrieval system, without written permission from the publisher.

Printed in the United States of America

For information:

www.marriage4alifetime.org

Destiny House Publishing, LLC
www.destinyhousepublishing.com
P.O. Box 19774 - Detroit, MI 48219

888.890.4555

Table of Contents

Acknowledgements

We have put in a lot of love, effort and time into writing this book. We prayed over this book and asked God's guidance. So it is fitting that we acknowledge Him first. Thank you Lord for your word and the awesome privilege of writing this book.

Thank you for the testimony that you handed us to share with others. We praise you for all that you have done, all that you are doing in our relationship and all that you are going to do. We are looking for more because we know you as the God of abundance. Thanks for your love and mercy. We are forever indebted to you for salvation and all the benefits that have come with it.

Secondly we would like to acknowledge our children who have shared their parents in ministry and in the process of writing this book. Jake and Keila: as you are starting out on your journey for a lifetime of love, always remember to keep God first and each other, as the next priority. You have a strong foundation. Build on it. A good marriage takes lots of work. Don't stop working.

Kyria, Charity, LaTina, and Christopher: Marriage is a serious commitment. Be sure of your potential spouse. You've seen the example that we have walked before you. So do not compromise. And be the spouse you want to attract.

We acknowledge our parents, Rivers & Nadirah Moody, John & Beatrice Walker, Mamie Rudolph, Andrew & Gwen Davis. You guys are a blessing. We thank God for your support and love.
We acknowledge our Granny aka Little Mama. We love you. Thank you for your example of commitment in 50+ years of marriage with Granddad before he transitioned.

We acknowledge our host of siblings and their spouses. We love you and consistently pray for you and your marriages (and for those of you who are not married yet, we pray for your future unions). May your marriages flourish for a lifetime.

To the entire Greater Works Family Ministries of Detroit, you guys are the best. We love and appreciate

you. You are by far the best church on the planet.
Blessings and peace to your marriages and
future marriages.

Special thanks and love to Joceline Bronson who
worked so diligently to help us get this book in its
second printing to press.

Special thanks to Cleaver & Susan Davis who allowed
us to use your story and are now leading our One Flesh
Marriage Ministry.

Acknowledgements to our friends and colleagues for
all your prayer and support:

Ken & Arzella Baker, New Covenant
Bennett & Angela Bradley, Valley of Blessings
Mark & Sherri Bryant, Women of Purpose
Linda D. Harris
Dave & Jeanne Kaufman, Holy Life Tabernacle
Doretha McBride, Kingdom Life Fellowship
John & Minnie Hardy, Make Us One Ministries
Zachary & Danielle Osborne
Casey & Nina Pringle, New Testament Holy Church
of Jesus
Shelia Rawlings
Lepoleon & Claudia Thomas
Larry & Torrona Tillman, New Destiny Christian

Church
Alfred & Janice Townsend, Real Ministries

To all our other family members and friends, we love you too. But there are just too many of you to name. We pray that you have marriages that mirror heaven.

Introduction

This book is written for all those who are divorced, have considered divorce, are in the midst of a divorce, and even for those who are happily married. There is a common thread that runs through the first three groups. In contemplating divorce, there is a level of pain and betrayal that many have shared. It is like nothing else that one has ever experienced.

The emotional pain is so intense that many think they may never recover. There is such a great level of hopelessness and isolation that occurs, as a cloud of darkness hovers over one's life. On the contrary, once restoration occurs, an exuberant and refreshed feeling overcomes you - it is the ultimate high. You become intoxicated with love. You may have never known that type of joy ever existed and never thought you could ever experience it. How could God love you this much? It's as if you wake up to love for the very first time.

We hope that this book will cause you to awaken to

the love of Christ and to the love of your spouse. God will do only what we allow Him. If you are in the midst of despair and doubt about your relationship, we want to encourage you to take a look at Hope. Jesus is the Hope of Glory.

No situation or circumstance is out of His reach. If we will turn it over to Him, He will overturn it for us. Our thoughts are not His thoughts, neither are our ways, His ways. So it doesn't matter if we can't see how He will do it. We just need to trust that He can. People allow human relationships to change their relationship with God. Your faith in God must be strong enough to combat negative influences. Even when you are undergoing a problem within a "natural" relationship - it should never interfere with the "spiritual" relationship you have with God, the Father. Nothing should be able to separate you from the love of God.

The word of God is true. He is holding us responsible to keep His word and our vows. As children of God, we are to be covenant keepers. It is so easy to dismiss the promises that we made to God when tragedy hits our relationship. Often we excuse ourselves and say, "God will understand" and the phrase "until death do us part" becomes nothing more than just a cliché added

to the wedding ceremony. But our covenant keeping God has a bigger plan.
He wants us to stand when adversity hits our marriage. If we choose to stand like Daniel did in the lion's den, we will see the awesome power of our God. He will stop the mouth of the devourer. The roaring lion will not be able to consume us. Trust in the unfailing God for a better marriage. It is His will and ultimate desire for you.

Finally, to those who are enjoying marriage, it is our desire that you remain on this path. We pray that you will adhere to the concept of divorce proofing your relationship. Keep the enemy out at all costs.
Learn from our mistakes and the expensive mistakes of others. You don't have to go through everything to learn it. You will find that experience is not the best teacher but the hardest teacher. Continue to love one another and always expect more in your relationship; there is always room for growth. And remember to strengthen and encourage others.

Chapter 1

The Way We Were

I spent the first two weeks in tears. I cried everyday.
I felt angry, hurt, betrayed, alone and desperate all at
the same time. I heard the words I had suspected for
months-my husband had been unfaithful. What was I
going to do? It's embarrassing that my first thought
was very much the same as an unbeliever. DIVORCE.
The world automatically chooses divorce when there is
a breach in the relationship. As a believer, why did I
immediately consider from the
world's list of alternatives? God had already
eliminated divorce as an option for His children. Yet,
I felt I had no other choice. I never even considered
healing.

When believers are in pain, we often respond by the flesh; gravitating to the sin nature. The old man is revived and we do not operate by the Spirit. We go with what we know - the familiar. That can be dangerous when what we know is limited. The Word clearly says destruction occurs, when we lack knowledge.

I felt the pressure to do something, immediately. So I did what I thought everyone expected, I asked my husband to leave. I thought this would be the only way to face the pain of infidelity. On the contrary, I felt like someone had reached inside of me, ripped my heart out and was now handing it back to me. I was devastated and confused. I didn't know what to do.

How could I trust my husband? Who was this man to whom I had given my life? He was the one I trusted most. He was my friend and confidant. We had been through so much. He knew my deepest longings and secrets. How could this happen to us? We were both Christians and we loved God. I had so many questions and I thought leaving him was the answer. Maybe, I would "*feel*" better.

Feelings lie in the soulish realm of man. They are not dependable. That is why the scriptures remind us to lean not to our own understanding. We have a commission to walk in the Spirit. Did any of this relate to the storm that was going on inside of me?

I (Oscar) was in shock. Yes I was the "perpetrator". I was the one whom the enemy had used. But I was hurting, too. I felt - used. I felt weak and foolish. The enemy had used me against myself. What was I thinking? I longed to turn back the hands of time. I wanted to change everything. This one foolish decision seemed to cost me everything. Would we ever recover? I had brought so much damage to the relationship. This situation brought back all the insecurities I had ever felt in my life. I loved my wife, as much as I knew love. But how did I create such a mess? How would I ever live this down?

The answer seemed simple and obvious - I wouldn't be able to live it down. My sin was too much to bear. So I felt that we ought to cut our losses and move on. She really didn't deserve this and I didn't deserve her.

Since we decided divorce was best, we called the divorce attorney; the estimate was $800. The expensive price tag caused us to seek another direction. We didn't want this marriage in its present state. We felt trapped. It would cost us too much to separate and too much to stay together. We fell on our faces to God. He took us on a journey toward finding Him. The journey was agonizing; because we believed in our hearts that we had already found the Lord.

It was a necessary and painful process and along the way, He found us. Deep in our hearts, we wanted to be found. Today we are glad that we got through it, because we are better for it. Abortion of this painful process would have been costly.

Discovery Zone

Two questions entered my mind. Was God looking for me? And didn't He know where I was? The answer to both questions was a resounding, "Yes!" He knew exactly where I was, but He was looking for me to grow up in my relationship with Him. He found me right where He knew I was - in this mess of a marriage. He wanted to change it all for me. He ministered to me. He loved and comforted me. And then I began to find Him.

Our relationship dramatically changed. We spent many more hours talking together. I searched the scriptures voraciously. An intimacy developed, that I never knew we could have. My savior and I fell in love. He began to teach me about His kind of love - a love that reaches past betrayal and failure. It was a compassionate, unconditional love that I had never known. God's love and mercy were so pronounced, that it breathed new life into me. He spoke directly to my pain. And He gently walked me through each stage of healing.

At one point, I (Crystal) began to sink into a pool of bitterness. I was drowning in my own selfish ambition of vengeance. I wanted my husband to pay for what he had done to me. He needed to reap some of this pain and I wanted to witness it. I knew it was wrong. But my flesh wanted gratification. I became the accuser of my husband. My character now reflected the old crafty one. God spoke to me and said, "His sin is no bigger than your sin." "What??!" I was appalled. I was at least trying to live saved. He wasn't even trying. How could God even compare the two of us?

We were nothing alike. I considered his sin as one on the big list. His sin was up there with murder and incest. I, on the other hand, was a loyal, faithful wife, committed to my marriage. I was the "good" Christian.

The Lord allowed me to stew in my polluted thoughts for a while. He eventually spoke to me again. This time, He spoke to me about the pride and self-righteousness in my life. It was difficult because I didn't want to deal with my own sin.

I wanted God to talk to me about my husband's sin. I wanted Him to say, "You poor thing. You deserve so much better. This man was not good enough for you." But He wouldn't. Every time I went to Him in prayer, He kept dropping this mirror in front of my face. He knew what I needed more than I knew myself. It all seemed so unfair.

This yoke-destroying, burden-bearing Lover of my soul threw me a lifeline. His love is incredible. He loved me while I was broken, wounded and flooded with insecurities. I felt ugly and worthless. Yet, He was kind and faithful throughout the entire ordeal. He intended to change my self-image. He wanted me to see myself through His eyes - not my own.
Before the fall of my marriage, I never knew God as my friend. I always thought of him as this great big judge with an enormous gavel, sentencing my every deed. I came to find out this picture was misconstrued. These thoughts were directly from the master deceiver.

For the first time in my life, I heard God say to me, "I love you." Yet, I felt like such a failure. And God was wooing this total failure to Himself. How could He

love me? Didn't I have to be neat, clean, and spotless? This whole "I love you" thing messed up my perception of God. I knew that God so loved the world and that He loved us in general, but I never thought He loved me specifically. How could this be? I was such a screw-up and it was visible by looking at my marriage. God don't you see this? He did see it. He saw the end of it. He saw
what He was going to do.

For it is in our weakness, that He is made strong. Without a doubt, His strength is perfect. In the midst of my filthiness, God continued to pour out his love on me.

This avenger of my soul bottled up each and every tear. He wanted to perform a wondrous act in my life; He would later cause those tears of sorrow to be turned into tears of joy. God's plan to mend this marriage was already in action. As much as He abhorred this sin that caused me so much pain, He still loved the one guilty of the sin, my husband. This man was a backslider and an infidel.

But the Lord, my God, loved this fallen man with a passionate and burning love. He had a history of loving fallen souls. This plan included two fallen souls - this man and his wife.

I (Crystal) wanted to trust the Lord and completely surrender my life to Him because He really cared about me. But it was difficult trusting anyone during this season of my life. My life was wrapped up in my marriage.

So once it cracked, I struggled with trusting anyone. God, in His infinite wisdom, delicately walked me through this phase of my healing. He was patient and understanding. His loving kindness drew me to Him and caused me to change my mind. God knew I needed my mind renewed and He knew that I needed to hope and dream again. My spiritual vision improved. Soon, I began to believe that God could heal our relationship.

I started a new relationship with the Lord. Interestingly enough, it was also the beginning of a new relationship with my husband. The Lord was handling us, molding us, changing us. This was the beginning. And we were the vessels that He had handpicked to use. God's word became life to us. We found out that all things "really" do work together for our good. Satan had a plan to destroy our relationship. God had a plan to draw some glory out of it. Thank

God that He always wins.

This began to resemble God's original plan of redemption for mankind, the plan of reconciliation. In God's original plan, Christ was wounded for our transgressions. And He died so we could live. The scriptures say, that it pleased the Lord to bruise Him (Isaiah 53:9). The crucifixion of Christ was master planned by the Father. He orchestrated the whole scenario.

Each character was carefully selected. And in the end, God was glorified. The sufferings of Jesus were prepared. Each stripe was intended. Much like our own marriage situation. It pleased the Lord to bruise us. Why would God get pleasure out of our pain? He is omniscient. He knows the end of a thing at the very beginning. He knows that pain produces promise. This whole aching event was necessary. It was part of the script.

"A woman when she is in travail hath sorrow, because her hour is come: but as soon as she is delivered of the child, she remembered no more the anguish, for joy that a man is born into the world." St. John 16:21.

With every contraction, she is closer to her deliverance. Her pain seems unbearable; but it is temporal. Our situation was similar. It seemed like we would not make it through the process but our just God would not put more on us than we could bear and we made it.

In that same way, we are bruised for purpose. God intentionally considered what was needed to build our testimony. And He began to set the scene in motion. Our marriage had been built on a shaky foundation.

We entered into covenant not knowing God or what being married required. Our house was built. Except the Lord build the house, they labor in vain that build it. The Lord had to *re*build our home. He tore down the shaky, ragged foundation that we had laid. We had to be broken. We had a contaminated love. We needed new hearts that could embrace God's pure love.

We didn't really want to divorce each other. We just thought we did. It was our way of stopping the pain. Of course, this was just another lie from the deceiver.

Divorce only intensifies the pain. Divorce can never heal. Healing never results through the choice of sin. Healing comes through choosing Christ.

How could anyone "really" want to divorce? We

wanted other things (joy, peace, companionship, etc.) and we thought that divorce would allow us to get them. All of these things come through relationship with Jesus Christ.

A Work In Progress

I began to work on myself. I (Oscar) did too. Neither of us was wiser as to what God was doing with the other. I (Oscar) would spend my lunch hour thinking about the situation - because I was too distraught to eat food. I hated who I had become. Everyday, I would cry out to God to remove my reproach. It's like you go through your daily life wearing the giant scarlet letter. You try to remove it but you know that you are guilty.

Only God can remove the reproach. Proverbs 6:32-33 says, "Whoso committeth adultery with a woman lacketh understanding: he that doeth it destroyed his own soul. A wound and dishonor shall he get; and his reproach shall not be wiped away." It was awful that I had committed this trespass against my wife. Worse than that, I sinned against God. It is a terrible thing to sin against God, especially after you have come into the knowledge of the truth. I was being chastened and I could not wipe away my sin. It would take God to cleanse my wretched heart. I needed a right spirit to be renewed in me.

This was the most difficult time of our marriage. Everyday I dreaded going home, but in my heart I wanted to be there. I just needed things to be "normal". I didn't have anyone I could talk to. I, the "violator" was suffering just as much as the victim, my wife. I continued to cry out to God as my heart broke every time I thought about this mess I made. God was speaking to both of us. I (Crystal) would go through these bouts where everything was okay and then the next day I would be infused with anger. My husband never knew what would happen when he came home. I hated the way I felt and I wanted him to feel sorrowful. I wanted him to tell me that it should have never happened but with the right amount of remorse. Although he apologized over and over again, his remorse was never enough. My heart was still hard. I struggled with the picture of myself that God chose to show me - it wasn't pretty. He wanted me to change who I was.

The adultery proved to be a symptom of a larger problem - we had problems with love and it stemmed from our backgrounds. We learned religion and not true relationship so we never became skilled at how to receive love. As a result, we were deficient in loving others. We thought we loved God, but the Bible outlined his lovers as those who obey His word. We both fell short.

The love we had for God was based on emotions; we had to learn how to truly love Him. In order to do that, we had to be willing to open our hearts to Him. Honesty would lead us to love.

I (Crystal) cried out to Him and said, "I want to know you, Lord." My prayers became more focused on my relationship with God. I stopped praying about what I felt should be the "unforgivable sin".
The Lord put me on a new path.
I began to discover the nature of Christ - love that did not fail. I had a desire to learn how one could love like this.

The children of Israel committed adultery several times. They chased after other gods but God continuously forgave them. What kind of love is this? This kind of love was foreign to us. This is a love that does not keep a record of the wrongs but offers a new mercy with the break of every morning.
The people that mocked, spit on, and crucified Jesus, were the same ones for which he chose to die. We were the sinners. Yet, He (who was without sin) died in our places. Jesus cried out from the cross, "Father,

forgive them for they know not what they do." How kind; Jesus did not want us to get what we deserved.

He asked the Father not to hold our sin against us. Then a thought crossed my mind, "What if we did know? What if my husband knew the damage he would cause when he committed adultery? What if I knew that I was storing bitterness in my heart? Even still, Christ saw the larger picture and knew, despite what we thought, we still lacked knowledge. His death and resurrection was applicable in every part of our lives. We just didn't understand it.

Our Gentle Redeemer died for us while we were unaware of His plan. He was asking that my husband and I do the same for one another - die to the flesh. Death is never pleasant. However, we longed to witness His resurrection power in our marriage. So a death was necessary. Our flesh needed to die. Pride, selfishness, lust, and unforgiveness - all of it had to be killed. This would only come from the power of the Holy Spirit. We could not continue to operate with the secular mentality that divorce was an option.
We needed to learn a new vocabulary: forgiveness, restoration, and reconciliation. More importantly, we needed to learn how to trust in the Lord with our whole hearts. Death to our flesh would mean that Christ could increase. When He is increased, He is

glorified. We could bring glory to God by allowing
our sinful flesh to die. This meant we would have to
follow his beautiful love story of redemption.
We had to learn how to be loved by God. Only then
could we display agape love toward others.

Nevertheless, we had a lot of repenting to do.
Obviously our way did not work, so we were going to
do it differently this time. We started with a clean
slate. My husband and I both submitted to God and
said, "Lord, your way and not our way." We decided
to apply the word in our lives because we made up in
our minds to really live it. We reached the place
where the Lord could cause victory to come forth in
our lives. We were in a position where we agreed with
each other and with God. The power of agreement,
however, is still underestimated in Christianity. It is an
explosive tool when two hearts unite and agree for
God's purpose.
God changed our hearts, lives, and world. We both
wanted to be in God's will and we wanted to be in
love again. So we allowed God to rewrite our love
story.

Today, I am a submissive wife. I love trust and
respect my husband. He is my best friend. I write
him love letters each anniversary telling him how I
would marry him all over again. We hold hands a lot

and spend Fridays dating each other. He still sends me flowers, opens car doors, and pulls out my chair. And he is a man after God's heart. For that I am most grateful.

I (Oscar) have learned to be honest with my wife, something I hadn't known before. She is my queen. I enjoy spending time with her. She laughs at my jokes and she makes me feel good about who I am. She is my lover and lifetime friend.

God has turned our mess into a message. The Word of God says the He can do exceeding abundantly above all that we could ask or think. So, we continue to ask for more in our relationship; and He continues to take our marriage to another level. Our marriage is abundantly blessed. And to think, we almost tossed it away. Today, we speak this message of hope across the country. We thank the Lord for interrupting our fleshly plans.

There's more good news. We are not the only ones with such a testimony. There are countless others who have experienced the same power and victory in their marriages. We weren't the first and we certainly will not be the last. God is the same today, yesterday, and tomorrow. He is still in the business of restoration and He wants to show himself strong on behalf of those whose hearts are perfect toward Him. Won't you give Him your heart?

Chapter 2

A 3-Fold Cord

How do couples get to the point of divorce? Usually there has been a weakening in one or both of the individual's relationship with God. A healthy marriage is based on a triangle with Christ being the head and the husband and wife are at the base.

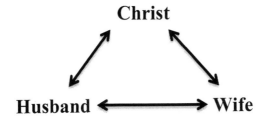

The relationship that we have with God will reflect in the relationship we have with our spouses. The horizontal relationship (relationship with spouses) is clearly a reflection of the vertical one (relationship with God). Our relationships will remain as strong or weak as our relationship with the Lord.

When we have the Lord Jesus Christ at the heart of our relationship, it will thrive and produce. A threefold cord is not easily broken. And the devourer cannot have easy access to the relationship. Being devoted to Christ and constantly spending time with Him makes it difficult for the enemy to wreak havoc. But when the three-fold cord has been worn and the relationship is lacking, the enemy has a gate.

We must realize that we cannot do anything by ourselves but only by Christ. The Captain of our souls knows exactly what we need. When we dismiss His presence, we will certainly suffer the consequences.

My wife and I suffered. We had confessed Christ as our Savior but He was not at the center of our relationship. All of our actions were based on the flesh and not on the word of God. Even the words we spoke to each other were disrespectful and harsh. We were spiritually empty. The transformation in our attitudes and actions had not yet manifested. We had to allow the Holy Spirit to have free course in our lives.

In actuality, God's word becomes the fuel for our relationship. It is only through a life hidden in Jesus does anything make sense. Two beautifully adorned human beings show up at the altar. These weak and imperfect people come with baggage.

Lots of baggage which include fear, insecurity, anger, deceit, pride, greed, lust, cynicism, manipulation, unforgiveness, control, and lies among other things. Remarkably enough, these are the things that kill marriages.

Sin in our lives will destroy our marriages. God has set this thing up. **When we work on our flesh, we work on our marriages.** He is able to keep us from sin if we stay connected to Him. If I kill lust in my members, I also kill it in my marriage.

Therefore, adultery has no place in my relationship. So Christ is crucial. Marriage is spiritual. It is a lovely illustration of the Bridegroom and His precious bride. Ephesians 5:22 admonishes husbands to emulate the love that Christ has for His bride. Chris loved His bride so much that He laid down His life for her.

I (Oscar) have learned to die for my bride. I protect her and provide for her. I love her without condition and I bless her with the desires of her heart. I am walking with her as I look to Christ's example.

I (Crystal) praise my husband. I respect and honor him as the church honors Christ. I do not speak words hastily because he is my lord. I delight in submitting to his headship. He is my beloved and we are in this covenant relationship for life.

Marriage is good and it works. God designed it. It was all His idea. A marriage that works is one that trusts God, believes, and obeys His word.

But it doesn't come easy. It will take effort. Contrary to the popular cliché, strong and healthy marriages are *not* made in heaven. They are made on the earth, in the daily routines of life. There will be no marriage in eternity. Marriage is simply for a lifetime. It is unrealistic to believe that marriage would be without challenges - no problems, no disagreements, no disappointments, and no trials. A truly healthy marriage is made on earth in the midst of frustrations and hard times. Christ makes the difference.

With the power of God, a three-fold cord is not easily broken. We need everything that God has to offer us in our marriages to help them remain strong. In that, we must follow His word. If God is the center of the marriage, the covenant is sealed. God is looking to fulfill His promises for us but it is our responsibility to live according to His Word. It is impossible to fight a spiritual battle by the flesh. The scriptures encourage us that is not by power, nor by might, but it's by the Spirit, that we win. A marriage with Christ at the helm is destined to succeed.

If you do not have Christ as the center of your life and marriage, you can accept Him right now. The scriptures say in Romans 10:9, 10 that , *"If thou shalt confess with thy mouth, the Lord Jesus, and shall believe in thine heart that God hath raised him for the dead, thou shalt be saved. For with the heart man believeth unto righteousness; and with the mouth confession is made unto salvation."*

Say this prayer with us: Heavenly Father, in the name of Jesus Christ, I recognize that I am a sinner (or backslider). I confess my sins to you and I believe that you sent your Son to die on my behalf. I also believe that He was raised from the dead on the third day.

I accept the work that He has done on the cross for

me. I ask that you forgive me for my sins and cleanse me from all unrighteousness. Thank you for loving me in my sin. Come and live in my heart forever. I believe that you are the God of life. Give me a new life in you.

I also invite you into my marriage. Guide me with your divine wisdom. I can do nothing without you. Give me understanding. Instruct me in the ways of righteousness. Let your glory be revealed in my marriage. In Jesus' name I pray. Amen.

Chapter 3

Covenant Keepers

Our faithful Lord is a covenant-keeping God. He never breaks covenant with His bride and He expects that we do not break covenant either. In Romans 1:31, a covenant-breaker is listed with those who had committed fornication, murder and even haters of God. He says that they which do such things are worthy of death. This is pretty strong language. God wants us to understand what a serious offense it is to break covenant. When a couple divorces they are breaking the covenant of marriage. We hurt God when we break covenant.

Divorce had been said to be a worse experience then the death of a spouse. The pain of divorce is violent. When you have two individuals who have become one, the ripping away is much like that of having your tongue stuck to a steel pole in sub-zero weather. You lose a part of yourself, trying to pull away from the other person.

That's why God says that divorce is treacherous. It does such damage to the heart that it affects all other relationships, including our relationship with God. Unless we allow the Lord to heal us, we become stifled in our ability to love. The residue of divorce hinders our love walk.

We become suspicious, jealous, fearful, untrusting, doubtful and guarded. These are not the fruit of agape love. I Corinthians 13 says, *love suffers long and is kind; it envieth not; it vaunted not itself, is not puffed up. Love does not behave itself unseemly, seeketh not her own, is not easily provoked, thinketh no evil; Love rejoiceth not in iniquity, but rejoiceth in the truth; beareth all things, believeth all things, hopeth all things, endureth all things. Love never fails.*

"Father, Father, why have you forsaken me?" These are the words that Jesus echoed as He was being crucified. Christ felt the agony of divorce and He knew the heart-wrenching pain of feeling abandoned. For the first time in history, he was separated from the Father. The penalty of sin required that we be forever divorced from the Father. But Jesus paid the price for us on Calvary. He became sin for us and He was deserted because there was a violation of man's covenant with God. Jesus suffered the excruciating pain of divorce so that we would never have to experience it. Yet, we choose it over and over again.

Christ loves his imperfect bride unconditionally. When one loves from a covenantal love, they love despite situations. We know that God's love is characterized by His sacrifice. He lost so that we could gain; He died so we could live. He gave so that we could receive. It seems that we get all the benefits of this one-sided love. Yet, He hopes and wills that we would love him back. Even if we don't, He still loves us. There is not a requirement for us to return his love. *While we were yet sinners, Christ died for us. Romans 5:8.*

His love is unconditional; yet, it is interesting that we, who are created in the likeness of Christ, have not yet learned to love unconditionally. The flesh does not want to suffer or sacrifice. Yet suffering is a part of the salvation package. The scriptures say that in order to reign with Him, we must suffer with Him. And they that live godly shall suffer persecution. The Lord tells us not to think it strange when the fiery trials come to try us as though some strange thing happened to us (I Peter 4:12). The sad thing is that not only do we think it's strange; we think that it is outrageous and unnecessary. We refuse to walk through this short trial to give God glory. So, we abort the process. The Lord forewarned us about the suffering we would have to endure; and the crosses we would have to carry. Yet, the minute suffering begins, we are ready to throw in the towel, If we could take a stand for Christ, He would receive a worthy offering of what He has purchased for Himself.

The Bible says, that when you vow a vow, defer not to pay it. That simply means that we have to keep the word that we speak. God requires that our word is reliable. If we speak it out of our mouths, we ought to honor it. In this evil hour, it is scarce to find true men and women of their word. We can barely keep a promise to return a call, more or less, anything of more significance.

On their wedding day, a couple stands before the minister and witnesses and casually state that they will love, honor and cherish, in sickness and in healthy for better or for worse, "until death do us part".

Unfortunately the point of disagreement becomes the death of the marriage. The vows would be more accurately translated *"until he gets on my nerves"* or *"until there is not enough money"* or *until she commits sin"*. God designed the marriage to last for a lifetime. Even if it is not spoken in the marriage vows, God still expects that marriage would last for a lifetime. Covenant is important to Him. In Joshua chapter 9, we find the story of the Gibeonites, Israel's neighbors. They heard about Joshua and how he defeated Ai and Jericho. They knew they would be next so they developed a plan. If they could somehow get Joshua to make a covenant with them, they would be fine.

They began to question how to make Joshua enter a pact with them. They knew they could not simply ask him. Someone thought, "Let's trick him." Their thoughts must've continued, "But won't he kill us if he finds out that we are deceiving him?"

"Yes, but it's a chance that we will just have to take. Either way, we stand to die." So they got some dry molded bread, put old sacks upon their donkeys and gathered some old, tattered wineskins. They went all out for this charade. They got old clothes and shoes and told Joshua they came from a very far country. They asked him to make a covenant to not harm them and they would be his servants.

The men of Israel were a little suspicious, they asked, "How do we know that you are not our neighbors?" The Gibeonites continued their deception. "We took this bread fresh and look; now it is molded."

The Bible says that Joshua asked NOT counsel at the mouth of the Lord and he entered covenant with them. Three days later, he found out that these wily men were his neighbors.
The people of Israel were outraged. But Joshua 9:19 reads, *"We have sworn unto them by the Lord God of Israel therefore we may not touch them."* God would not allow Joshua to touch these people because of the covenant he made with them. Our God requires that we always keep our word.

For those who think this to be unfair, God always makes a way of escape for us. Had the men of Israel asked the Lord's guidance, He would've revealed who these Gibeonites really were. They didn't ask and so they found themselves in a situation they didn't want to be in. God made them keep their word. They would've died had they went back on their word.

God is so interested in keeping covenant that this situation returns generations later in the book of Samuel. David had a problem because of the covenant that Joshua made with these same people. In II Samuel 21, David had been praying about the famine in the land that had been there for 3 years. The Lord said, "It is on account of Saul and his bloodstained house, it is because he put the Gibeonites to death."

Saul was in rebellion. But because Saul was a man who didn't honor God, he didn't honor covenant. Look at the judgment it brought upon the people. When we dishonor covenant, it causes judgment to come upon us. David had to do something to eradicate the judgment that was upon the land. He asked the Gibeonites what could be done to restore honor back to their relationship.

After David renewed the vow with the Gibeonites, II Samuel 21:19 reads, God answered the prayers on behalf of the land. God will bless us if we choose to restore instead of replace.

Many of God's people are suffering because they broke covenant. God withheld the land from the children of Israel because of a broken covenant. We will not receive the full blessings and promises of God until we become covenant keepers. Satan's job is to break the covenant. God will do everything in His power to preserve the covenant. His word means everything.

Let's examine the covenant made with the Gibeonites again. Not long after Joshua made the covenant with them, he had the opportunity to prove whether or not he would keep the covenant. Joshua 10:3 reads, "So Adoni-Zedek king of Jerusalem appealed to Horam king of Hebron and unto Jarmuth and unto Jachia king of Lachish and unto Debir King of Eglon saying come up unto me and help me that we may smite Gibeon for it hath made peace with Joshua and with the children of Israel."

These kings decided to make war against Israel because of the covenant. God is so concerned about covenant that in this battle He caused the sun and the moon to stand still. There is no other time history where this happened. God will ensure victory when we honor covenant.

"I know the thoughts I have toward you. They are thoughts of peace and not of evil, to prosper you and to bring you to an expected end." God is speaking to His people. We can stand on His word. It may seem like punishment to remain in your covenant. But there really is a plan to bless you in the midst of it. God knows what He is doing; we just need to trust Him. If we allow Him, He will deliver His promises in our lives. The power of the cross is available to us today.

When we choose divorce, we choose a curse. Divorce is not the will of God for us. The blood that Christ shed was designed for the suffering that would happen in our lives. He subsequently gave us power over all the powers of the enemy. We as believers should never embrace what God says he hates (Malachi 2:16).

He has broken the curse of sin and death in our lives. Jesus does not desire that any of us should experience such pain. He has already suffered for us. He is able to redeem our sins if we simply yield them to Him.

Chapter 4

Mending Broken Pieces

Just as there is life after death, there is hope for a failing marriage. God is all-powerful and there is nothing too hard for Him. The God who has power over death is able and available to resurrect our marriages. The requirement on our part is that we believe.

Christians believe that God is able to heal the sick from cancer and even raise the dead. But our faith in His power does not extend to heal marriages. We tend to believe that our God is capable of doing anything else except heal our relationships.

We believe that the one who created marriage does not value it enough to save it. But, God, who is a restorer and a reconciler is halted only through unbelief.

Our Lord called us to be ministers of reconciliation and he is able to mend any situation that we may bring. Unfortunately the church has bought into the secular excuse that our differences are irreconcilable. But if God is omnipotent, how can this be true? The scriptures remind us in Matthew 13:58 that Jesus could not do mighty works in the city because of unbelief. If we will just believe, nothing shall be impossible for us. Trusting in the infallible God will allow us to see the miraculous.

My wife and I have seen many marriages restored in the body of Christ. Even after the breach of divorce. We know that earthly judges do not have the final say, but God does. God's desire is to restore and renew our lives, so when we take our broken situations to Him, He is able to mend them. Jesus said, "The Lord has anointed me to preach good news to the poor, to set at liberty the captives, to heal the brokenhearted, and to release from darkness the prisoners." The Lord is willing to heal us.

Wounded relationships need to be cast at the altar of

the Lord. These damaged relationships require the skilled hand of the Living God. When we attempt to carry our own burdens we err because they are much too heavy for a mere man. The Lord has the power to turn our mourning into joy and ashes into beauty.

We must recognize the need for the Mender and know that He has an earnest desire to repair our breaches. He is the Potter. We are the clay.

A songwriter once penned some lyrics about God as the Potter. The song encouraged us that we don't have to stay in our messed up situations, the Potter desires the opportunity to repair the breaches. And he has everything we need.

This song is a message of hope to the hopeless. The Finer will do away with the dross that troubles us. He will bring forth a vessel that is fit for himself. Come just as you are battered and bruised and He will begin putting those pieces back together.

But how does the mending begin? He starts at our faith. You must start with a faith that says God will do it for me. Most of us know that He can do it. The question that we are often faced with is, will He do it? We must raise our level of faith to match God's power.

We must have faith large enough to accommodate a large enough God. Faith speaks God's word and it causes God to move on our behalf. Faith is what we really hope to see when we can't see anything. It's what we speak when nothing makes sense.

The Word of God will only profit us if it is mixed with faith. A wounded marriage is an opportunity to unleash faith and allow God to perform the miraculous. If we lack faith, we will find it impossible to please God. Our lifeless words become self-fulfilling prophecies. Comments like "My marriage can't be saved", "It's too late for us", or "Even God can't help my spouse" will stop God's power because doubt always cancels faith.

How do we get faith? Faith cometh by hearing and hearing by the word of God according to Romans 10:17. We must hear God's word over and over again concerning our situation. We must go out of our way to get the word. God's word gives life and hope. We live in a time where the word is readily accessible. Wisdom is crying in the streets. We simply need to activate it.

It is important that during this mending or healing process, we hear God's word of restoration and healing. We must hear it until we believe it.

God will cause faith to move us to the next level of wanting Him to move on our behalf. Jesus asked many people before He healed them, "Will thou be made whole?" That question is echoing through the ages. "Do you want to be healed?"

Healing begins with the individual. The marriage is secondary. Forgiveness is the springboard toward our total healing.

It begins with the choice to agree with God's Word and it requires that we bring our brokenness and lay it at the feet of Jesus because He is our Healer. When Jesus went to the cross, He did not only bring salvation, but provided physical, emotional and spiritual healing; and He made it available to us. The bride must be whole when Christ returns. All spots and wrinkles have to dissipate. What will we say to our Lord, when he had made a way for us to be free from offense?

As believers, we should not elevate our offense to the point where we refuse to forgive. There is no name or situation that is higher than the name of Jesus. We need to come to the "heart" knowledge that **all** have sinned and fell short of the glory of God. We have made mistakes and offended others intentionally and unintentionally.

Because of that, there is a requirement to forgive on our part. If we have never sinned, if we have never needed anyone to forgive us, then it is not necessary that we forgive others. But because, we are born in sin and shaped in iniquity, we all need forgiveness.

Forgiveness involves releasing the offender from the offense. It says to the offender, "You will not receive what you justly deserve. You are released from this offense as if it never happened." That's what Jesus did for us and He requires that we offer this to others, including our spouses.

The amazing thing about forgiveness is that it not only releases the offender, but it goes a step further and releases the offended. Once we have made the choice to forgive, we are refreshed.

Forgiveness takes a present offense and puts it in our past. We are not subject to the torment of remembering the wound anymore; and we will be able to walk in peace and wholeness. Unforgiveness will hold you captive to the offense. We think about it. We speak about it and even hurt about it. But once we free the offender, we free ourselves.

It is only when we hold on to unforgiveness, that we forfeit our peace. Unforgiveness causes our hearts to become hard. A hard heart can never please God, except to repent. We cannot say that we love God and hate our brother or choose to be bitter at our spouses. God loves His creation and asks that we love others the way He has loved us and the way we want to be loved.

Every time there is an offense in our marriage, there is a challenge present. The challenge causes us to declare what we really believe.
If we call ourselves "believers", we must ask ourselves, "What is it that we really believe about Christ and His death?" When we are offended there is an opportunity to rise above the fleshly response to render evil for evil and show what Christ taught us: To love the unlovable, to overcome evil with good, and to bless those who persecute us.

It is so easy to agree with the Word of God when we are not faced with challenges. However, if we belong to God, we will always be challenged. We will always be faced with the challenge in our lives to agree with the Word of God through obedience. We can constantly say that we believe it is wrong to hold a grudge until we are faced with forgiving someone.

Most of us believe that we ought to forgive others when they sin against us but when we become the offended person; the Word is not challenged in our lives.

Our values are demonstrated in our actions not just what we speak with our mouths. Forgiveness is the choice process that expedites healing.

What are the practical steps to forgiveness?

- **DO NOT REHEARSE THE OFFENSE TO OTHERS.**

One of the most dangerous actions when you have been offended is to replay the situation to others. The offended person should not go from listener to listener recounting the story of how he/she was violated. This is equivalent to ripping a scar off of a healing wound. You are saying, "I want you to see that I am bleeding. Look at what the offender has done to me." It is an attempt to gather an army of sympathizers. We want them to say we are justified in our anger. This encourages us in our bitterness and causes others to look down of the offender.

This is one of the risks of talk shows and court shows. Their television programs drain the slightest chance of reconciliation from the relationship. One spouse airs his/her marital problems to a group of strangers (who are unconcerned about their relationship or wellbeing).

The audience is there to be entertained by the couples' weaknesses and relationship breach. This same audience will walk away 30 minutes later, never to be seen again. Now the hurting couple has to live with everyone else knowing their problems.

In many cases, one of them will side with the audience against their spouse. However, we believe that when others become involved it defeats the "forsaking all others" principle that applies to marriage.

Wisdom will not allow us to air our marital disputes to a host of others. Family and friends are no exception..

It is unhealthy to tell our loved ones about the offenses our spouses have caused. When we have forgotten, our loved ones still remember. This makes the reconciliation process more challenging because our loved ones will always have an opinion. If we give energy to their biases, we will have a harder time reconciling the marriage.

Our family members will tell how they disagree and they will even challenge our willingness to reconcile. Not only that, but we damage the reputation of our spouses even if what we are saying is true. If we put ourselves in the place of the offender, how much would we tell?

What if we were wrong, would we want everyone to know about our offense? Love says that "as hurt as I am, I will not talk about to others until I am healed, even then it will be with wisdom." Let the words of

my mouth…be acceptable in thy sight.
Psalm 19:14.

Even if our spouse is walking contrary to the Word.
God still requires that we honor our marriage
commitment. "Let this same mind be in you, which
was in Christ Jesus." Christ surrendered his right to
be right. We must do the same. He was sinless but
became sin for us. We, his bride, have been
unfaithful, time and time again. And Christ still loves
us and He never rehearses our offenses to others.

He tosses them into a sea of forgetfulness as far as
the east is from the west and remembers them no
more. We, who are created in the image of Christ,
have no right to slander our spouses. In our tongues,
we hold the power of life and death. We must not
misuse the power that God has given us because it can
become bitter water - condemnation
and gossip. Out of our belly ought to flow rivers of
sweet, living waters - hope, life, and encouragement.

• MAKE A CONSCIOUS DECISION NOT TO MEDITATE ON THE OFFENSE

Another tool in satan's arsenal is *tormenting thoughts.*
Satan will bring up the offense and say, "See how
wounded you are? You were so mistreated and you did

not deserve it. Why did this happen to you?" If the enemy can cause you to feel sorry for yourself and turn all your thoughts internally, he will disrupt the healing process in your life.

Your thought will eventually turn to accusing God. Self-pity is a terrible sin that is rooted in pride. As we pity ourselves, we begin to voice within ourselves that we do not deserve such treatment and we wonder why God would allow something like this to happen to us. We think our faults are not as wrong.

This is an eroding thought process that will eventually cause us to elevate ourselves above God. Pride, bitterness and unforgiveness will eventually turn our hearts against God. We try to justify ourselves and in turn, we think that God is unjust. That is why it is important to rebuke impure thoughts immediately.

When we replay the offense in our mind, it becomes poisonous to our spirit man. It is better to think about God's goodness.

Our mediation needs to be on His grace, mercy and compassion toward us. Think about how God is healing us and how much He loves us. We cannot allow the enemy to get a stronghold. Therefore, it is essential that we do not allow ourselves to meditate on the offense because it refreshes the wound. If we continue to contemplate on how we are to so misused and abused, it becomes our reality. The Bible instructs us that as a man thinketh in his heart, so is he. We have to decide not to allow the enemy to have his way any longer in our lives.

We must free ourselves from this bondage of torment. Philippians 4:8 says, "Whatsoever things are true, honest, just, pure, lovely, of good report, if there be any virtue or any praise, think on these things. The promise of God is that He will keep us in perfect peace whose minds are stayed on Him. *Let the…meditations of my heart be acceptable in your sight.*

• ALLOW TIME FOR HEALING

The mending of a marriage is very much like the healing of the body; it takes time. But time does not heal all wounds. It is the healing blood of Jesus. And that requires healthy doses of forgiveness. Nevertheless, the process of healing, between a sickly relationship and a whole one, demands time. If the wound is deep, then healing needs to go deep. If the process is hurried for the sake of the offender, then the healing process will be superficial and true

reconciliation will not occur.
However, one cannot confuse the choice of
forgiveness with feeling the pain of the wound.
A person can choose forgiveness long before he or she
actually feels whole again. We must remember that
forgiveness is **not** an emotion. It is a choice. The
offender must allow the wounded person time to heal.

• FORGIVE AGAIN

What if the offender does not have a heart of
repentance, should we still forgive? As many times as
the offense occurs, we must forgive. We are
challenged to rise to a level of virtue that resounds 70
times 7. Have we sinned against God more than
once? Have we ever struggled with the same sin over
and over again?

We must forgive as much as we want forgiveness.
However, forgiveness is separate from the process of
restoration. Restoration in a marriage can never occur
until there is true repentance.

If the offender denies responsibility, does not stop the
offense, or is impatient about the process, restoration
should not occur because Godly repentance is the only
way to restoration.

True Repentance

II Corinthians 7:10-11 reads, "For godly sorrow worketh repentance to salvation not to be repented of: but the sorrow of the world worketh death.

For behold this selfsame thing, that ye sorrowed after a godly sort, what carefulness it wrought in you, yea, what clearing of yourselves, yea, what indignation, yea, what fear, yea, what vehement desire, yea, what zeal, yea, what revenge! In all things ye have approved yourselves to be clear in this matter." When the repentance is fleshly or emotional, the sin will reoccur. But godly sorrow will manifest itself in the seven virtues aforementioned. First, the offender becomes careful about his actions because he does not want to further afflict or offend. He becomes sensitive to the pain of the wounded and does everything in his power to ensure healing. The offender cannot rush the healing process. Nor does he tell the offended spouse to *just get over it*. Carefulness is very important.

Clearing yourself means ensuring you have mended every area of the situation. The offender's position should be one of wanting to clear himself at all costs. When Jesus entered into Zacchaeus' home, Zacchaeus began to repent of his sin. He said if I have taken anything from any man by false accusation, I will restore him four-fold. Zacchaeus was clearing himself. Whatever sin we may have committed, we must choose to clear ourselves. That means that we will do whatever it takes to get in right standing with the Lord.

That is not always easy but it is always right. Indignation is anger directed at the enemy of our soul. We should become angry at sin instead of our spouse. Indignations says that I hate evil. We should get upset at the enemy because he has taken advantage of us but we are no longer ignorant of his schemes (II Corinthians 2:11). The offender recognizes that he or she was taken advantage of by the deceiver and so mad at the devil that he/she will not allow Satan to take advantage again.

The **fear** of the Lord is to depart from evil. It is also the beginning of wisdom. So this fear means that you come into a spiritual understanding of the offense.

The offender does not want to violate his relationship with God. He/she values the mercy of God and seeks to avoid the very appearance of evil. This person has such a reverence for God that he/she will not allow their good to be evil spoken of. The offense, with a heart of repentance, should cause you to be so concerned that you not want to commit the sin again and you do not want it to even *appear* as if you are committing a sin.

The offender has such a vehement desire and zeal, which is a strong desire and passion for righteousness. The offender becomes passionate in his desire to deter others from the mistake he has made.

He does not mind speaking out against what he has done. He will warn and exhort any that he feels may fall in the same ditch. However, the offender must be sensitive to the offended spouse (carefulness). The spouse may not be ready to share the testimony with others.

II Corinthians 10:6 reads that we must have a readiness to revenge all disobedience, when your obedience is fulfilled. **Revenge** means to punish. As the violator or offender, I am willing to accept the punishment for my disobedience without trying to justify myself. I am justified by faith. But I am willing to suffer the repercussions of my sin, with full knowledge that God is able to turn my situation around.

In all these things we have approved ourselves to be clear in every matter. So we can see the fruit of repentance. However one should not be alarmed if these fruits don't manifest all at once. God can and will work on the offender, if you continue to pray. Satan may break your relationship, but God will mend every broken piece and it will be as if it was never broken.

Chapter 5

It Ain't Over

It was a beautiful fall day. The bride was impeccably dressed and the groom stood handsomely awaiting his "good thing". We performed the ceremony and it was beautiful.

The bride's name means "grace" and the groom's name means "holding or cleaving." Today they are holding on to the grace of God. We had the honor of marrying this lovely couple that had been in counseling with us for a year and a half. We took our time because they had been married once before to each other. Unfortunately, divorce had infected their relationship. They had many problems that needed to be worked through. This was the day that God would be glorified. The devil thought he had them. He thought it was all over. But God was able to restore the relationship.

The God of restoration brought this union back under His divine plan. Isn't it interesting, that just because a judge (a man) says that a union is over, we believe it? We forget the power of our God. We think, "Well they're divorced now. It's over!" It's not over! Creation is not more powerful than the Creator.

My wife and I have sat in divorce proceedings with other couples. We go with them as an act of faith in standing for their marriages. Our presence says that we do not believe that the marriage is over, no matter what the judge says. We spend most of the time praying for God's intervention. Usually there is such a strong spirit of bitterness in that courtroom and the atmosphere is so cold and harsh that it feels as if a death has occurred.

Every time the gavel hits, I imagine God's heart breaking. "Let no man put asunder what God has joined together." And the devil smirks as the judge asks the couple, "Is there any way that this marriage can be reconciled?" One spouse says yes and the other says no. The divorce is granted. Isn't it remarkable that both have to agree in the wedding ceremony but in the divorce proceeding, one can get out without the agreement of the other? What is the point of the question if they do not have to agree? We believe that this is a scheme of the enemy. He wants us to confess out of our mouths that our God is powerless. "No judge, there is no way that this marriage can be reconciled." The devil looks at God and says, "These are your children. They do not even believe in your power." He laughs. When we talk to couples about standing and waiting on God, the response we often get is either, "I am moving on with my life" or "It's too hard!" First of all, for whom is it too hard? It's certainly not too hard for God. If we cast our cares upon Him, we won't carry the weight of it. So it can't be too hard for us. Secondly, how can a believer move on with his life when our lives are in Christ? It's in Him that we move, live and have our being. Just imagine for a moment that God has a divine plan.

He wants to reconcile you so that you can tell others. Would you be willing? God is looking for men and women that will stand for righteousness in this dark hour.

Postmodernism is a theory that is used in our American society and it means that nothing is absolutely true and everything is relative. But postmodernism cannot be the standard for the believer. Jesus said, "I am the Way, the Truth, and the Life. No man comes to the Father, but by me." We must accept God's way. Christ is absolutely the truth. We, as Christians, cannot do what every man thinks is right in his own eyes. We will not yield the peaceable fruit of righteousness. We should not rely on our own understanding. Rather, we ought to submit our lives to the will of God.

There are people all over the world, who love God and their spouses and believe God to reconcile their marriages. We have seen many couples reconciled after a divorce. There was one couple that was remarried after having been divorced for 15 years! Truly God was glorified.

The couple we mentioned at the beginning of this chapter was divorced for three years. Some walls had to be torn down. But we had to get them to believe that divorce was not their end. Nothing had been written in stone. Divorce is not irreversible. Divorce is only as final as our hearts are hard. If we are willing to wait on God, He is able to redeem our shattered relationships.

The problem with us is that we never want to wait on

God. And if we think that it is going to take any length of time, we'd "rather not" wait on God. Patience and her perfect work are thrown out the window, because we are an anxious people.

Often times we wind up in the next marriage as unhappy as the first. Why? Because we thought we could choose better and faster than God. Not only that, but divorce is a spirit and if we embrace it, we carry that spirit into the next relationship.

Waiting produces character. God must not only change the wayward or offending spouse but He must also change the waiting spouse. God sees the two as one, so he will not deal with one spouse without dealing with the other. He is preparing the waiting spouse to die to the flesh. If the Holy Spirit is not working within the waiting spouse then he or she can become a hindrance to reconciliation. Self-righteousness, pride, selfishness, bitterness, and vindictiveness can begin to sprout.

"But God told me to divorce, my husband." We've been told this a few times. How is that possible if God hates divorce and prohibits it in His Word (Malachi 2:14-16)? Every word from God must align itself to the written word of God. God never ever speaks contrary to His word. We spoke covenant to

God and He speaks covenant to us. His covenant is from everlasting to everlasting. His covenant is for an eternity. Death is the only thing that can legally separate us. Is God changing his mind? Is He saying, "Don't worry about the vow you made before me?" Hardly! God does not change, people do. Divorce is against everything that God represents. His character is one of love and unity. How could He tell us to do something that He defines as treacherous? Marriage is for a lifetime and should only end where there is a physical death not when we feel like we cannot take "it" anymore or when a judge in a divorce court declares it to be over.

As a Christian you must understand that Satan is on a mission. He comes to steal, kill and destroy – that's it! If we could just wise up, we would see Satan as the deceiver that he is. Our eyes must be open to his devices. Divorce is one of Satan's most widely used weapons against believers. He tries to make us think that it is God's tool. Divorce's destructive nature could never be the plan of God. The Lord said, "I came that you might have life and that more abundantly." God would never create such an underhanded device to bring harm to His children.

But what about the exception clause?! Doesn't God give us a way out in certain circumstances? What does the word of God say? We have researched scriptures to find out the heart of God on this issue. Every man must be persuaded in his own mind.

Below are the scriptures on divorce in which we were confronted.

Malachi 2:14 For the Lord, the God of Israel, saith that he hateth the putting away: for one covereth violence with his garment, saith the Lord of hosts: therefore take heed to your spirit, that ye deal not treacherously.

Matthew 19:3-9 The Pharisees also came unto him tempting him and saying unto him, Is it lawful for a man to put away his wife for every cause? And he answered and said unto them, Have ye not read, that he which made them at the beginning made them male and female. And said, for this cause shall a man leave father and mother, and shall cleave to his wife: and they twain shall be one flesh? Wherefore they are no more twain, but one flesh. What therefore God hath joined together, let not man put asunder. They say unto him, Why did Moses then command to give a writing of divorcement , and to put
her away? He saith unto them, Moses because of the hardness of your hearts suffered you to put away your wives: but from the beginning it was not so. And I say

unto you, whosoever shall put away his wife, except it be for fornication, and shall marry another, committeth adultery: and whoso marrieth her which is put away doth commit adultery."

Mark 10:11-12 And he said unto them whosoever shall put away his wife, and marry another, committeth adultery against her. And if a woman shall put away her husband, and be married to another, she committeth adultery.

Luke 16:18 Whosoever putteth away his wife and marrieth another committeth adultery: and whosoever marrieth her that is put away from her husband committeth adultery.

Romans 7:2-3 For the woman which hath an husband is bound by the law of her husband so long as he liveth, but if the husband be dead, she is loosed from the law of her husband. So then if, while her husband liveth, she be married to another man, she shall be called an adulteress: but if her husband be dead, she is free from that law; so that she is no adulteress, though she be married to another man.

I Corinthians 7:10 reads and unto the married I command, yet not I, but the Lord, Let not the wife depart from her husband: But and if she depart, let her remain unmarried or be reconciled to her husband: and let not the husband put away his wife.

I Corinthians 7:39 reads the wife is bound by the law as long as her husband liveth; but if her husband be dead, she is at liberty to be married to whom she will; only in the Lord.
What will we do with all of the scriptures? Will we rip them out of the book or choose to ignore them? Clearly God has outlined to us, his heart concerning divorce.

When interpreting the will and principles of God, they can never be based upon one passage of scripture. A common theme throughout the Word of God needs to be found. When one's heart is open to hear truth, God will speak. His voice should not be ignored. If He desires to speak to us and He does, we owe Him the respect of listening and taking heed to His word.

Maybe you've already had a divorce. What do you do now? Perhaps you've already married someone else.

Repent of the divorce and denounce the spirit of divorce from your present marriage; and then stay in that marriage for a lifetime.

If you are divorced but not remarried, It's not too late for you. You can begin afresh. First repent. Ask the Lord's forgiveness and pray that He will soften your heart to His will.

Understand that there is **no condemnation** to them that are in Christ Jesus, who walk not after the flesh, but after the Spirit (Romans 8:1). While God hates divorce, He loves those who are divorced or have been divorced no differently than anyone else. Divorced people are NOT second-class citizens. We have all sinned and stand in need of God's grace. God loves you unconditionally.

Secondly, just because you come into an understanding of God's word does not mean that you will suddenly want your spouse back. That will take time. Certainly you don't want the marriage in its original state, you want what it can become. Allow God to make your heart pliable. You want His divine will and purpose for your life.

However you must choose to stand for your marriage. How does one stand? Draw on the promises of God from His word. Read the Word for healing, encouragement and strength. Reestablish your prayer life. Initially, you will find that most of God's words to you will be about you and not your spouse. Surround yourself with other believers and people who will support your stand.

You will have to spend minimal time with those who may think you are ridiculous; because they do not understand and may try to discourage you.
He that walketh with wise men shall be wise: but a companion of fools shall be destroyed (Proverbs 13:20).

Eventually God will give you instructions on how to handle your spouse. You must pray that your spouse will have a heart for reconciliation. God will give you specific directives on how to win your spouse back.
It cannot be done through manipulation or control. Allow the process of change to come forth freely and completely by the Spirit.

Stay encouraged by the fact that God has restored and is still restoring numerous marriages and He is not a respecter of persons. What He does for one, He will do for another. He wants to do it for you. Activate your faith. Your marriage isn't over.

Chapter 6

The Unforgivable Sin

If you were to ask believers, "What is the unforgivable sin?" Most of us would respond, "Blasphemy of the Holy Spirit". But ask us when we have been wounded and at the brink of divorce. Our response might change. For too many of us, it is adultery, abuse, addictions, abandonment, incest, or a host of other ills. The unforgivable sin becomes that offense that causes our hearts to be broken.

Jesus saith unto them, " Moses, because of the hardness of your hearts, suffered you to put away your wives: but from the beginning it was not so (Matthew 19:8)."

Here, Jesus is talking to the Pharisees. They had asked him under what conditions can we divorce our wives. He said, "none." They continued, "Then why did Moses allow us to divorce?" Jesus responded, "Only because you would not forgive. But God never allowed divorce." Men's hearts are hard only because men choose not to forgive.

We make up our own conditions. When in actuality, God never told us that we could hold unforgiveness. The scriptures name the unforgivable sin of blasphemy of the holy Ghost.

The Bible talks about the unforgivable sin of blasphemy in relationship to God administering forgiveness to us.

We do not have a right to say that we do not or cannot forgive. Because it is a requirement of our salvation. Since God forgives us, we have to release others. Mankind does not have his own "unforgivable sin" category of things that he won't forgive. God sets the rules. Our finite minds are unjust at best, therefore we must operate under God's specifications. Since God is the authority, we cannot set personal standards in our marriages or any other relationship in which we will or will not extend our mercy. In order to have the abundant life that He has promised, we must follow His plan. When we are wounded, we mistakenly think we can operate in the flesh, instead of allowing God to be in control. We execute judgment on our spouse, yet we want God to have mercy on us. It is the insanity of sin that causes us to operate so blindly.

Since our spouse operates in *the sin* that we deem as unforgivable, we choose to divorce him or her. Once we divorce them, we try to justify ourselves, but we are operating in opposition to God's Word. When the Word clearly says that God is the one who justifies us. God requires that we take care of others" needs first, and then our needs will be met.

An unforgiving heart will always operate against God's Word. As a result, today Christians have a higher divorce rate than secular society. Our hearts become evil because we do not believe God to reconcile our marriages. Mostly, we don't *want* to believe God because we want retribution. Every time we experience heartache, the flesh has an opportunity to live or die. At most times, the flesh is raging. It is alive and well and ruling our lives. In fact, the rising divorce rate is evidence that our flesh is winning.

How can we justify disobedience to a Holy God? Christians who hold on to unforgiveness, sometimes get caught up in rendering evil for evil. The Lord told us to overcome evil with good. We must abort our sin nature and take on the character of God.
If we do not, the sin of unforgiveness will remain in our hearts.
What do we do with the "70 X 7" scripture? Aren't we to forgive the offender again and again? Is not the entire ministry of salvation based on forgiveness?

Furthermore, the word of God says that if we do not forgive others that we would not be forgiven. So, in reality, unforgiveness becomes the unforgivable sin.

To label a spouse's sin as unforgivable is to deny God's power. As we open our mind and our hearts to the will of God, we will find that there is hope for our marriages. We will find that God is a healer. He is a repairer of the breaches. He is more than able to do the unattainable and unimaginable. But it requires that we begin to reach outside of societal norms and into the will of God.

We will have to begin to expect the impossible from the God who specializes in miracles for impossible situations.

Several years ago, my husband and I were guest speakers at a marriage conference. This bitter and angry woman came up to us and told us her story. Her ex-husband was an unbeliever and she was a Christian. She said he did not provide for her and the he was mean and wicked. They struggled while they were married; so she eventually divorced him and married someone else.

Her ex-husband had recently gotten saved. He was totally changed. He now had a good job and was doing quite well. This made her angry. She asked us "Why couldn't he have done that while I was married to him?" Our question to her, "Why didn't you wait for God complete his work"? Her flesh made a decision that cost her more than she wanted to pay. And even though she was at this marriage conference with her new husband, she was still miserable. She was in bondage to her bitterness. She should have trusted God to make her way.

Nevertheless, we as imperfect people make some crazy decisions. She should just repent, forgive and find joy where she is.

Does forgiveness always constitute reconciliation? Not necessarily. However that decision should not be determined by our sinful flesh. We must pray and submit to the leading of Christ. We can never know what is best for us but God always knows. Flesh always chooses opposite of God.

In the case where there is a battered wife or abused children, a time of separation may be needed. If the husband is seeking professional and spiritual help, there is hope for reconciliation. However, if the abuser doesn't see a need to seek assistance, reconciliation cannot occur until there is a noted change. However the wife must still forgive her husband. She can be separate from, forgive him and wait on God for a change.
We have seen couples reconciled under almost every situation. We have seen the drug-addict set free from his addiction.

We have seen the angry batterer delivered from his rage. We have seen the porn addict and adulterer liberated from their sexual bondage. We have seen a couple reunited after the wound of incest. Truly the heart of the king is in the Lord's hand. He is able to change every sin-filled heart.

Chapter 7

From Despair to Repair

"We are troubled on every side, yet not distressed; we are perplexed, but not in despair."
II Corinthians 4:8

The Greek word for perplexed is aporeo. It means to be at a loss, or in doubt. The Greek word for despair is exaporeomai. It means to be utterly at a loss. Paul is saying that although we may feel exasperated and doubtful about the challenges we face, we are not without hope. Surely Jesus is the Hope of Glory. In verse 9, he says that we may face persecution, but we are not forsaken, Jesus promised never to leave us.

Therefore although conditions may cast us down or we may be going through difficult situations, we still are not destroyed because greater is He that is in us that He that is in the world. Even when we feel like we cannot press on, we must look to the Word of God for the end result. Our God has caused us to triumph in Christ Jesus. When there is a breach in the relationship, our hearts bleed because our marriages mean so much to us. When hardship comes it pushes us off balance. But there is no relationship, challenge, or situation that supersedes the power of our God. He wants to work in us and through us.

Many marriages have been built on faulty foundations; therefore, they crumble at the slightest breeze or wind. The Lord does not want us to sit in a puddle of despair. We must get up; dust ourselves off and begin the rebuilding process. Before we can rebuild the walls of our marriage, we must examine the walls and assess the damage.

In Nehemiah 2:13, Nehemiah went to view the wall of Jerusalem. He needed to assess the damage done to the wall before he could rebuild so he looked around at the ruins of the walls and saw the places where it was broken down before he began to rebuild.

We must examine the walls of our marriages to see

where and how the enemy has broken in and why he was able to do so. At this point, we tend to miss it or don't realize the next step taken is the most crucial.

In marriages, the couple may see the need to do better and attempt to do it but what they may not realize is that it cannot be done by man's strength.

If we depend on our own strength to change we will always fail. A spouse may propose a list of things he will and will not do to help bring for the change. For example one may say that he will not drink, she will not nag, or that he will spend less money and begin spending more time with the family.

We want to do it, but we find that we don't have the power. Ultimately we find ourselves back in old comfortable habits and the marriage is still suffering.

We cannot deal with symptoms; we must deal with the root of marital problems, Begin by asking hard questions: how, what and why. Then you can uncover the cause.

If one of the spouses in the marriage is suffering from drug abuse, the couple needs to ask, "How did we end up in this situation?" They may discover a generational curse of alcoholism or drug abuse. When under stress, a person may revert back to old ways of handling stress. So if a job loss or sickness were to occur, this could trigger the inability to properly handle stress. The former drug user would revert back to old habits if his relationship with the Lord is not strong.

What caused the vertical relationship with God to weaken? Disillusionment or discouragement could have set in after a job loss. Perhaps the spouse felt as if God was not there for him.

Why was the stress handled with drugs? The individual must be confronted with this question. He must know why he chose drugs. He needs to identify his future options and eliminate some things from his present list of alternatives.

Assess the damage to the relationship. Is it in areas of trust? Evaluate how both spouses feel and decide that the damage is not irreparable.

Going back to Nehemiah, after he assessed the damage to the wall, he became sorrowful because of the people and the wall's condition. Similarly, we must be remorseful about our situation to the point where we desire repair. He also began to pray for direction. While this may seem obvious to some, as humans, we usually react first, then we pray. We must learn to pray first so we can seek the heart of God. Nehemiah recognized the character of God. He said that God keeps covenant with his people. We, too, are in covenant with God. Our marriages represent covenant.

Nehemiah repented of all personal and corporate sins (Nehemiah 1:6) *"I confess the sins we Israelites including myself and my father's house, have committed against you."* When Nehemiah prayed, he was not self-righteous. He prayed for sins he and the other Israelites had committed. When we pray for our spouses we must realize that we are sinful as well and our sins need to be recognized.

Even though our spouse may have sinned against us, we are responsible to pray as one. We confess our sins together.

The offended spouse usually asks, "How have I sinned? My spouse was the one who was involved in pornography (or some other offense)." If we allow our hearts to be tender, God will show us. The heart is desperate and deceitfully wicked, who can know it? God knows what's in our hearts. The sin may have only manifested as a result of the behavior of the violator. In any case, repentance is in order. It keeps pride out of the relationship. What is Christ trying to teach us? If all things work together for the good of those who love the Lord and are called according to His purpose, then there is something of value that we must gain from these challenges. Intrinsic as any painful situation is the knowledge of how to avoid that situation. More than that, there is some rubbish that must be expelled from our minds and our relationships. This is a difficult fact to face. There is often a mirror in front of us when we face a crisis. Our natural tendency is to avoid the mirror and find someone else to blame - mainly our spouses. We must realize that often both parties contribute to the tearing down of the walls. Self-justification will only slow down the process of repair.

Nehemiah also reminded God of his promises. "Remember the instruction you gave your servant Moses, saying „If you are unfaithful, I will scatter you, but if you return and obey my commands, I will gather you and bring you to a place that I have chosen."

God has made many promises for our lives and relationships. He said He would bless us with every blessing. He said that He would give us the desires of our hearts. He said that the seed of the righteous shall be delivered. He promises us peace, joy and His undying love. There are thousands of promises in scripture. We have to remember God's promises and remind Him of His promises. God hastens to perform His word. We must keep His word in front of Him. "Lord, you promised..."

Finally, Nehemiah requested specific help to begin the process. When you are in need of support and guidance for your marriage, don't be afraid to ask for help. There are people who have been where you are now and they can help you get through the obstacles. In the multitude of counselors, there is safety. Just because we are going through something, does not mean that you are in sin. It could mean that God is trying to teach us or impart something into our lives. If we learn it, the experience produces some value.

If we don't learn it, we are destined to repeat it. Isn't it disheartening to know that the children of Israel had a less than 2 week journey to the Promised Land, yet it took them a toilsome 40 years?

Throughout the entire time they never learned how to be grateful. They continued to murmur and complain.

We have to evaluate the distress that hits our marriage relationship. Ask God, "What should I have learned? What should I have gained out of this?"

There are five principles that are essential to rebuilding.

• BOTH PARTIES MUST BE ALLOWED TO COMMUNICATE OPENLY AND HONESTLY

Communication is key to the restoration process. However, the offender does not need to give details of the offense. The offended does not need to hear a play-by-play account. The offended may even ask for particulars, however it is not wise to comply. True communication requires that spouses talk through the root issues that plague their relationship, not the details of the offense. Focus on the real issue. For example, Anne and Lee Smith are recovering from an infidelity. The issue is not where the infraction was committed.

The root issue is where did the breakdown occur in the marriage? How did they wind up at this place in their marriage?

In our experience in counseling, we have found that most offended persons think that the offender has no rights. This is not true. The offender has a right to express himself and should be encouraged to do so.

Most times, the repentive offender is dealing with his own pain. If you are willing to work toward reconciliation, you must be willing to talk through the offender's pain as well as your own.

The offended cannot use this offense to hold over the Spouse's head to control or manipulate. Neither can it be used as a weapon to make the offender pay. "Vengeance is mine" saith the Lord, "I will repay." We cannot move on God's territory. He has not given the offender the right to punish the offended. If you've worked through the forgiveness process, you are not playing these immature games.
As a follower of Christ, our mandate is to pray for God's mercy toward the offender. This may not be possible initially but we can at least pray for a Godly response.

- **THE OFFENDER MUST BE SENSITIVE TO THE HEALING PROCESS OF THE OFFENDED SPOUSE**

At the same time, the offender must not push the offended. Just as we talked about true repentance, the offender must be willing to avenge himself. The correct attitude must be, „I will do anything to make this right." So if the offense was adultery, the offender must be willing to call home every time he is going to be late and account for additional time spent. The offender also must ensure that his spouse is emotionally secure and comfortable; and understand that trust has to be rebuilt. It is the responsibility of the offender to encourage the healing process. He must also pursue peace in the relationship.

Couples in healthy marriages may not have to go through such extensive measures, however once there is an offense, the relationship needs intensive care. These steps to rebuild are vital. These actions are presently necessary and will eventually cause the marriage to move into a healthy phase where they will no longer be required.

• DO NOT WALK ALONE

Walking alone is equally as damaging as telling everyone your business. It is dangerous to walk through this type of pain alone. The wolf loves the lone sheep. That lone sheep is easy to devour when he or she is not a part of the herd. When we are alone, tormenting thoughts are able to overwhelm us because our spiritual defenses are lower when we are wounded.

Therefore, it is necessary to have sound godly counsel to counter those thoughts from the wicked one. Ecclesiastes 4:9-10 reads, "Two are better than one; because they have a good reward for their labor. For if they fall, the one will lift up his fellow: but woe to him that is alone when he falleth for he hath not another to help him up." So in order to mend properly and expeditiously, we must have a trustworthy companion to walk us through this process.

A patient never goes into surgery without others because he cannot operate on himself. We have to select a person who is unbiased and willing to hold us accountable to the word of God. This person must be honest and compassionate and he or she should not be one that engages in spouse-bashing.

The person you choose to walk you through this process must be of the same sex. Relationships with people of the opposite sex at a vulnerable time can be risky. We are defenseless and cannot see as clear spiritually.

The enemy can and has devastated many marriages with "understanding friends of the opposite sex". Yet, these are men and women who are dispatched by the enemy to side track you from your path of restoration.

He or she can be a physical distraction from the will of God in your life.

These third parties usually are so considerate and kind that the bruised spouse becomes attached. Often the "distractions" are unaware that the enemy is using them. Their intentions are well-meaning. Mostly, they think that they are helping. Wisdom says avoid the very appearance of evil. If it resembles something evil, remove yourself from it. It doesn't matter how save this person appears. You must guard your heart with all diligence and walk in holiness toward those that are without the Lord. Your witness should not cause others to stumble. If there is not a same-sex godly individual to walk you through this process, you must pray that the Lord will send someone into your life.

- **SURROUND YOURSELF WITH PEOPLE WHO SUPPORT YOUR MARRIAGE**

Since this is a critical time in your marriage, you need to ensure that you are receiving strong Christian counseling regularly (weekly or biweekly). If you cannot afford counseling, you should find a mature married Christian couple with whom you **both** trust and agree.

It is not the exclusive right of the wounded spouse to

select such a couple. In working toward repair, both parties must feel comfortable confiding in this couple.

If this selection is one-sided, the repair of the relationship will be delayed and possibly aborted. Meet with this couple regularly and allow them to walk you through the process of reconciliation. They must be people who can challenge you when you are not walking in the Spirit. This couple should be mature in Christ and have weathered some marital storms themselves.

Beware: there will be some who will be against the restoration of your marriage. Handle them with wisdom. Know that they do not understand and ask them to pray for you (if they are Christians). However, do not seek counseling from them. Counseling from a couple who is not in support of your relationship can damage the marital reconciliation process.

You also need a cheer team. Get those that are supportive and meet with them regularly for prayer and encouragement. Choose only one or two friends with whom you can share your situation. You do not want to opt for those that are prone to gossip or who are bias. Everyone is not at a spiritual level to handle your situation properly. So be very slow to speak and extremely selective.

• DO NOT GIVE UP

Understand that you may hit some snags along the road to restoration and that it is not uncommon. There will be times that you feel like giving up, but hold on to your faith. As Christians, our mandate from God is to always walk by faith.

Put up scriptures on your bathroom mirror and other places around your house for encouragement. Listen to messages on faith and marriage.

Keep focus on the progress that you have already made and do not be afraid to celebrate good times in your relationship. This will help to keep you on target. Your family is at stake. Engage in warfare. You cannot afford to grow weary. Constantly pray for each other and your marriage. Jesus is faithful and He is on your side but you have to decide to stay on His side. God's word promises that we will reap in due season, if we faint not. Hide His word in your heart and do not give up. Remember true love never fails.

Chapter 8

From Top To Bottom: When Leadership Falls

Do leaders, pastors, bishops, and ministers fail in their marriages? Absolutely. Leaders are human beings so they do fail. All humans are subject to error. Leaders sin and when they do it can be even more devastating. One reason is because, when there is a problem in the marriage, it is seen on a wider scale. As a result, recovery can take a longer time; but God wants to display His power. This is a time to apply the Word of God that has been preached to others, this is a chance to allow God to restore, refresh and proclaim His glory. He wants to use you as a part of that process. If you are willing, He is able.

In scripture, there are many examples of fallen leaders. Look at King David. He was a wise and mighty warrior, yet he fell into sexual sin. Since his sin was not confessed, it took him deeper into sin. As a result, the king committed murder. We, as leaders, cannot think, at any time, that we are above God's judgment. Sin that is not confessed will always take you deeper than you expect to go. You cannot worry about what other people will say or think; you must be concerned about God's opinion. What does God have to say when He sees you commit the sin?

We must constantly say "I must be right before God." A heart of repentance always moves God.

Although God judges the sin of leaders, he will heal and restore them. God requires that we walk carefully before Him, constantly examining our hearts. Our hearts must remain pure before a Holy God. If you have a heart of repentance, God will restore you. Our hearts must cry, "Forgive us" daily, Paul says, "But I keep under my body and bring it into subjection lest that by any means when I have preached to others, I myself should a castaway" (I Corinthians 9:27). This is a standard by which all of us should live.

If there has been a failure in the leadership marriage, the leader should do the following:

Acknowledge the failure. Remember that failure is an event and not the person. God wants us to recognize and acknowledge our sins. Confessing it is an important first step. As leaders, we should not wait until our sins are exposed to repent. God loves a repentive heart. Repent to God, your spouse, your children, and your congregation.

Ask God for help in the reconciliation process. God will bring to light those things that need to be done. Ask the Lord for help but also seek help from outside sources. Counseling, a drug treatment program, gamblers anonymous, or an anger management class may be needed. Fall in love with Christ all over again.

Be Accountable. Whatsoever is asked of you, do it with all of your might and without hesitation. A leader must be accountable to a pastor, governing board or a group of pastors. A man that will not be held accountable is a dangerous man. His sin does not negate his anointing but neither does his anointing disallow correction to come forth in his life. God chastens those whom He loves. This one of the most encouraging passages in the Bible. We are all subject to chastening because God is just and He has established order in the earth.

Just as the wife must submit to the husband, leadership must submit to leadership. The prophet is subject to other prophets. In the past, leaders have left their denominations, or spiritual covering after a moral failure to avoid church discipline, but this in violation of God's principle of order. A leader should not resist those in authority to challenge him.
Humility proceeds restoration.

Leaders should not continue "their" ministry. A "business as usual" attitude denotes a selfish attitude and unrepentive heart. True repentance goes beyond a simple confession. There must be conversion - a true change of heart. This will allow time for healing to come to those families and the congregants involved. A true minister will do what is in the best interest of God's people. He is concerned about all of God's sheep, especially the "first sheep" (if he is a pastor), which is his spouse and children. Money, status or position should not be motivation for the fallen leader to resist chastening. There should not be haste to get back in the pulpit or any other arena of ministry.

Satan is against all of God's people. An attack against your marriage is also an attack against your ministry. A leave of absence or a sabbatical may be in order. Time should be taken to find out how the leader got off track. What defenses were let down to allow the enemy to come in?

Why were those defenses dropped? What could have been done differently? Ministers need to take time to rebuild trust with their family. They too have been violated by this breach.

Become proactive. Start doing what you did not do in the past. Avoid the sources that caused the breakdown in the first place. Pour more time into your family. Change your attitude and sow into your relationship. Fall in love with God and your spouse all over again. God will give you ideas and visions for your marriage as you become more proactive. Marriage conferences and workshops are seldom attended by leaders. Yet this is a strong protective measure against marital breakdown. Ministry marriages actually need more ministry than that of others. As examples, we need to preach only what we practice ourselves. Remember that your marriage is your first ministry.

Avoid over-commitment. After a leader is restored,

he must be careful not to over-commit. Leaders have to learn how to balance their time and energy in ministry. Consult and agree with your spouse about your workload.

Take weekends away with your spouse for renewal. My wife and I commit to getting away at least once every quarter.

The leader must also learn how to properly handle stress. I (Oscar) believe that leaders get into trouble by carrying too much on their plates. When we are feeling overwhelmed we need to talk to someone so that they can guide us. Stress not only kills a marriage but it kills people as well. High blood pressure, stroke, migraines, heart attacks, panic attacks, and many other diseases are the result of stress. We can find peace and tranquility in God who is the Prince of Peace.

Leaders do not have to fail. There are certain policies that should be put in place for every pastor or leader. Such policies not only preserve the presbytery, but keep ministering families whole and intact.

Leadership must have those to whom they share even the most personal part of their lives. They must be willing to be open and honest with these persons. If a minister is able to confide in another leader that he hits his wife, steps can be taken to help this man through his deliverance. Accountability is key to avoiding sin.

Women should counsel women and men should counsel men. This is a protective element. If this is not possible, a third party should be included counseling sessions when you are counseling those of the opposite sex.

Leaders should be careful of how they complement the opposite sex. Words must be carefully chosen as to not give the wrong impression. Many compliments have been misunderstood.
Never should a compliment regard the physical appearance.

Ministers must watch their hands. Leaders must be careful not to improperly touch someone. Embraces should be done with prudence. Leave space when hugging. If laying hands on someone, leaders should keep the hands above the shoulders.

Avoid touching the face and any part of the body below the shoulders. And never kiss any lay member.

Watch out for pride. Satan is always on the prowl.

We have to make sure that we safeguard against the attacks of the enemy. The number one weapon that he uses against leaders is the spirit of pride. As we walk in humility, we are unable to fall prey to his arsenal. Pride always comes before a fall. Pray for yourself. Take nothing for granted. Pray that the Lord will cover your marriage and protect you from falling into sin. I Corinthians 10:12 reads, "Wherefore let him that thinketh he standeth, take heed lest he fall."

Engage others to pray for you. Intercessors are a great covering. They are able to warn you of impending danger and pull down strongholds around you.

However, they cannot be blamed if you choose to sin. Sin is always a choice. God has given man an awesome free will.

Lastly, leaders should make sure that their spouses are visible in their ministries. Spouses should accompany them as much as possible. Allow your spouse to make a contribution to the ministry. An invisible spouse is easily erased from the relationship. A marriage is susceptible to permanent breakdown when a minister or pastor does not involve his mate.

Chapter 9

Never Broken Again

If your vow has been broken, God is able to seal it so that it is never broken again. When God restores something, it is regenerated to a state as if it never was broken. Yet we have to maintain whatever it is that God has done for us. Divorce or the threat of divorce does not ever have to touch your relationship again. Even if your union is strong and healthy, there are things you can do to divorce-proof your relationship.

HONOR YOUR VOWS

"Until death do us part." Keep your vows sacred.

Understand that the covenant that you made with your spouse included God. Eliminate the decision to divorce as an option. Commitment will cause a marriage to stand even when you feel love is lost. Stay true to your covenant. You will still have situations that arise in the relationship that will cause offense. However, you must decide to follow Christ's will and plan for your life.

Believe that your love and marriage are forever. People act according to what they believe. If you believe that divorce is not an option, you will do whatever it takes to make the marriage work.

If you believe that Christ is fully powerful, you will not belittle his death, burial, and resurrection in your life. You will see it as suffering for your sake and the sake of your marriage. Your choices will begin to align with the will of God.

NEVER THREATEN TO DIVORCE

My husband and I never us the word "divorce" as a threat to one another. That word is forbidden in our household. The scriptures say that life and death are in the power of the tongue. Words can release spirits and we will not release them in our marriage. We don't even entertain the thought of divorcing.

This was a problem in the early years of our relationship. I (Crystal) was the guilty one. At every little infraction, I would let the words fly off my tongue, without even considering the damage that I was doing.

Thank God for second chances. We have reclaimed our lifelong covenant and refuse to surrender it ever again. Our covenant is sealed. No matter what tribulation we may face, we will love each other through it. Divorce is not an option for us. This has made a big difference in our lives. It has brought security in our relationship with one another. We know neither of us is going to abandon the relationship. So our marriage ascends to another spiritual level. The same promise that God made the church, my husband has made to me, "I will never leave you nor forsake you. I will be with you always even until the ends of the earth." I, too, have made that promise back to him. We refuse to speak death over our lives. It doesn't matter what the offense, we know that we can work it out.

You must choose the same thing. Some people may be so insecure that they are afraid to commit like this to the relationship. They fear that it will give their spouse a license to roam or do whatever he or she feels. This is not valid. We have to ask the Lord for help in

breaking our old mindsets. Speaking life brings life.
Speaking death brings death.

LEARN TO FIGHT FAIR

We have to attack the problem and not each other.
Satan understands the power of agreement. His trick
is to get us to fight against one another. The wisdom
of God will allow us to pool our energy together and
instead of fighting against each other, we war against
the enemy.

The Bible says one will put a thousand to flight and
two, ten thousand. Our spouses are never our
enemies. Satan is the true culprit.

We are careful to assault the enemy of our souls. We
pray about the discrepancy and seek God's guidance.
We know that at any time we both could be wrong.
Communication, however, must be clear. For example,
I am upset because I need more household
support but I am not angry with you. Therefore focus
must stay on the need for more support and not on the
person's character. Calling the spouse names like lazy
and inconsiderate takes the focus off the problem.

Name-calling, yelling and bickering are immature
works of the flesh. Keep the conversation moving

toward healthy solutions. (Can you help by doing the laundry once a week, and the dishes twice a week?) Arguing solves nothing. If we do not stay focused on the subject at hand, we will try to bring up the past in our arguments. This is also unfair fighting. We often bring up the past to strengthen our argument. The past must remain in the past. *"...Forgetting those things that are behind, I reach for those things which are before... Philippians 3:13"*

Mature Christians do not use the past against their spouses. It is pointless to say, "Three weeks ago you said you were going to spend time with the family but, then you went out with your friends that same night." That is the past. It is more appropriate to clearly define what it is you hope to achieve. You cannot say you need more time without clearly identifying what your expectation is. Say things like "I would appreciate it if we could have family time once a week. On Saturdays we are usually all free. Will that day work for you?" Once you agree on a day, you should plan the activities that will be held on that day for the next month. You should also ask if it is okay to offer a gentle reminder if needed.

Proverbs 15:1 reminds us that *"A soft answer turneth away wrath: but grievous words stir up anger."* We must never render evil for evil but we must walk by the Spirit. We understand that the tongue is a dangerous weapon and it has ignited wars between nations.

We must learn how to bridle our tongues and allow the law of kindness to be found there.

Never forget that words are spirit. If we get lost in emotion in the heart of the moment, heavy damage can occur. At all times, we must remain levelheaded, so conflict can be minimized. It is important to understand each other's position. Try putting yourself in the other person's shoes and listen to their heart more than their words. Repeat what you understood the person to be saying.

Listening is a lost art. We need to listen intently and not try to think of what words we are going to say next.

The problem with unfair fighting is that some couples refuse to talk at all. The silent treatment is a divisive tool of the enemy and is not the will of God. If we walk in the Spirit, we will avoid using the tools of Satan. What sense does it make to walk around days and even weeks without speaking to one another? Clearly the plan of God is that we do not allow the sun to go down on our wrath.

He says be angry but don't sin in that anger. When we walk around explosively silent, we are sinning against our Holy Lord. The silent treatment represents an unforgiving and bitter heart.

KEEP ONE ANOTHER FIRST

No person (including your children) should come before your spouse. This is not to say that we are to neglect our children. Together we have a command from God to love, care, and provide for our children. But neither are we to neglect our marriage relationship for our children. Sometimes children are allowed to bring a wedge in the relationship.

These same children will grow up, marry, and become one with their own spouses. So one day they will be grown and gone. Keep your relationship with them in perspective.

Don't allow them to play one of you against the other. Couples must forsake all others and cleave to one another. In-laws, friends, and other family members must come second to the covenant.

No one should be allowed to voice his or her opinions about your marriage or criticism of your spouse. Family members should not be allowed to belittle or make jokes about your spouse. We need to guard our spouses from hurtful comments, so that others will not feel at liberty to cut down our spouses. Even your pastor and boss are both secondary to your relationship with your spouse.

This is a principle that some in the church have not yet embraced. This means you cannot favor what your boss says over your spouse. Your spouse's desires should come before that of your pastor. Honor one another. You will be surprised how others will respect your marriage.

INVEST IN YOUR RELATIONSHIP

As you begin to date your mate, it will take you back to the courtship phase of your relationship. Usually, that is the time when the relationship was exciting and pleasurable. We believe that dating is not an option or a luxury but it is a necessary effort. In order to reap the benefits of a joyous union, we must sow time into one another.

Date night is every Friday. We laugh, learn, grow, and even cry together. We have spent many intimate moments strengthening our marriage. We have visited museums (art and historical), carnivals, athletic events, movies, plays, dinner at a fancy restaurant, a picnic in the park, watched movies and many other fun activities. We are creating happy memories with each other.

You will be surprised at how your marriage is strengthened by such a simple act. Not only do we have a date night, but we also have weekend getaways, every quarter. Boy, do we look forward to those! It ignites passion into the union.

The lack of dating in your marriage can cause a dry, stale relationship. It leaves your bond vulnerable to the destruction of the enemy.

If babysitting is an issue, trade babysitting with another couple. You watch their kids every 2nd and 4th Saturday and they will watch your children every 1st and 3rd Saturday. Barter with a close friend or relative. In lieu of payment, agree to wash their car for a month, or some other thing in which you may be skilled.

Dating your spouse is not a chore. It is not meant as a punishment. Dating can be fun, adventurous, and fulfilling. Yet, it is one of the most difficult things to get couples to do together. The excuses pile up.

However, anything that is worth having requires a time investment. Approach it with excitement.

So sit down together and choose a day that is convenient for you both. Surely you can find one day out of seven to pour into your marriage. Dating will work wonders in your relationship.

DEVELOP YOUR SEXUAL UNION

Sex is the glue that binds you to one another. Dr. James Dobson of Focus on the Family Ministries has recommended that couples come together sexually every 2 to 3 days because it keeps your covenant fresh.

If there are some health concerns or worries about an unexpected pregnancy, schedule an appointment with your physician. Eliminate any situation that threatens your physical union, with your spouse. Buy a lock for your bedroom door, if privacy is an issue. If it's just been awhile, take a shopping trip for new lingerie. Talk about those sexual taboos that may haunt you and see what the scriptures say. God invented sex. He intended for man to fully enjoy his wife and vice versa.

I Corinthians 7:3-4 tell us that the wife's body belongs to her husband. And the husband's body belongs to his wife.

"Let thy fountain be blessed: and rejoice with the wife of thy youth. Let her be as the loving hind and pleasant roe; let her breasts satisfy thee at all times; and be thou ravished always with her love (Proverbs 5:18, 19). Celebrate marriage. Married sex is the best sex.

You don't ever have to go through the trauma of a marital breach again. It is finished! We don't have to re-defeat the devil. He is already defeated. We just have to walk in our authority as believers.

The blessings of the Lord maketh rich and addeth no sorrow. Enjoy the blessed union that God has given you. Take time to divorce-proof your relationship. You will find as we have, that God will do great things on your behalf. More than you ever could imagine!

Prayerfully, the spiritual truths in this book will help you to stand on the word of God. We have prayed for every reader of this book. It is our desire to see you grow in your relationship with God and with your spouse. The word of God is life giving.

Read the scriptures. Allow them to take root in your spirit. Hold on to your faith and trust in the Almighty Deliverer. His promises will come to pass in your life. We hope that this book will give you hope and encourage you in your marriage. May you forever be one flesh.

Chapter 10

Scriptures For Encouragement

Joel 2:25
I will restore to you the years that the locust have
eaten, the cankerworm, and the caterpillar, and the
palmerworm, my great army which I sent among you.

Romans 8:28
And we know that all things work together for good to
them that love God, to them who are the called
according to his purpose.

Proverbs 21:1
The king's heart is in the hand of the Lord, as the

rivers of water: he turneth it whithersoever he will.

Jeremiah 32:17
Ah Lord God! Behold, thou has made the heaven and the earth by thy great power and stretched out arm, and there is nothing too hard for thee.

Luke 1:37
For with God nothing shall be impossible.

Psalms 31:11
The Lord will give strength unto his people; the Lord will bless his people with peace.

Philippians 1:6
Being confident of this very thing, that he which has begun a good work in you will perform it until the day of Jesus Christ.

Hebrews 13:4
Marriage is honorable in all, and the bed undefiled; but whoremongers and adulterers God will judge.

Philippians 2:13
For it is God which worketh in you both to will and to do of his good pleasure.

Psalm 126:5
They that sow in tears shall reap in joy.

Luke 18:27
And he said, the things which are impossible with men are possible with God.

Psalm 30:5
For his anger endureth but for a moment; in his favour is life: weeping may endure for a night, but joy cometh in the morning.

Galatians 6:9
And let us not be weary in well doing: for in due season we shall reap, if we faint not.

Romans 8:18
For I reckon that the sufferings of this present time are not worthy to be compared with the glory which shall be revealed in us.

Psalm 115:11-12
Ye that fear the Lord, trust in the Lord: he is their help and their shield. The Lord hath been mindful of us: he will bless us; He will bless the house of Israel; he will bless the house of Aaron.

Jeremiah 31:16
Thus saith the Lord; Refrain thy voice from weeping, and thine eyes from tears: for thy work shall be rewarded, saith the Lord; and they shall come again from the land of the enemy.

II Corinthians 5:17-18

Therefore if any man be in Christ, he is a new creature: old things are passed away; all things are become new. And all things are of God, who hath reconciled us to himself by Jesus Christ, and hath given us the ministry of reconciliation.

Q&A

1. What if my husband/wife doesn't want the marriage? What can or should I do?

→ You can stand on God's Word. Prayer is a powerful tool. God wants your marriage restored. You can stand in agreement with the Lord for your relationship. He is able to heal. Nothing is too difficult for Him. Many marriages have been healed because one person chose to believe God.

2. My spouse has cheated on me. I don't trust him anymore. I know I must forgive. I want to but I don't. How do I forgive?

→ You must first *choose* to forgive. That has to be first and foremost. It doesn't mean you won't have angry feelings. But your choice must line up with God's word. The feelings will eventually follow. Whenever the thoughts come regarding the offense, you must pray for your spouse and not meditate on them. Read scriptures on forgiveness. Don't allow your friends or family to discuss the offense with you. You have made a choice to forgive. So begin to behave in accordance with your choice. Don't act as if your spouse owes you something for the offense. It is also a good thing to study scriptures on forgiveness. *He who covers and forgives an offense seeks love, but he who repeats or harps on a matter separates even close friends. Proverbs 17: 9*

For if you forgive people their trespasses [their reckless and willful sins, leaving them, letting them go, and giving up resentment], your heavenly Father will also forgive you. Matthew 6: 14

3. My spouse and I are working toward reconciliation. Do you have any advice for us?

➡ Congratulations! The best advice is to make sure that you are in counseling. The best and surest reconciliations work when there is a third party holding the couple accountable so as to not repeat the transgressions of the past. A good counselor will also make sure that you are not moving too slow or too fast in the process. He or she is able to objectively evaluate the relationship. So our advice is to get in counseling right away!

4. My parents are difficult to say the least. They are both elderly and set in their ways. My husband wants nothing to do with them because they treat him so bad. Is it wrong for me to expect my husband to have a relationship with them?

➡ It is kind of you to look past your parents offenses, because they are aging. You want to make sure that you have done right by them. That is understandable. However, a relationship works two ways.
Your husband cannot have a relationship with someone who doesn't want it. Not only is it unfair for you to expect your husband to have a relationship with them, but you have a duty to lovingly confront your parents regarding their comments and/or actions toward your husband.

5. There is a woman at my husband's job. I believe she likes him. I have told him about her on many occasions. He just pushes it off as if it's nothing. He thinks that I am wrong and he is not taking it seriously. I am very uncomfortable with the little things she does to get his attention.

➡ Spend time praying for her. And by all means pray that the Holy Spirit would open your husband's eyes. In the meantime, you and your husband need to seek counsel. It is good to advert problems before they occur. Be proactive. Because women know women and men know men. So husbands should be respectful and make adjustments anytime his wife is discerning that a woman has impure motives.
In the same way, a wife should honor her husband.

6. My husband is a good man. We have 2 children and have been married for 7 years. I am overwhelmed because total responsibility for the kids and the home rests with me. I discipline the children, feed, dress, and clothe them and help them with their homework. I do all the cooking, cleaning, and laundry. This does not include all the errand-running I am expected to do. I also work full-time outside of the home. I am physically, emotionally, and spiritually exhausted. Most of the time, my husband can't help because of his job or other church commitments. My question is "does God require all of this of me as the wife and mother? Am I over-reacting?"

→ A marriage relationship can only prosper when both spouses are active in the relationship. It is unreasonable to expect 1 person to pull the weight of the entire family. Do not ask your husband to help out *occasionally*. His help must be part of the routine. If your husband is unable to assist with the running of the household, you may need to leave your job to give full attention to your first ministry. Your children should also be given age-appropriate chores. You married to be a part of a team, not a solo act. Gently discuss this with your husband. If it does not produce any results, you need to get counseling immediately.

7. Is it possible to outgrow your spouse?

➡ The word outgrow means to grow out of or away from; to grow too large; as, to outgrow clothing; to outgrow usefulness. When you outgrow something, it means you have no more use for it. You will probably discard it or pass it along to someone else. It is not possible for a spouse to outgrow his/her mate. The covenant relationship establishes a durability clause. Marriage is a lifetime commitment.

We are thankful that Jesus, in all his glory, holiness, and power, does not outgrow his bride. He promises to be with us always, even unto the ends of the earth. If we have the mind of Christ, we cannot outgrow one another. Outgrowing a relationship is a secular concept. Its root is in the spirit of pride. Surely couples are not always on the same level spiritually.

But our charge is to become one in the relationship. And we have an entire lifetime to work that out.

8. I have recently heard you say that the husband comes first in the marriage before the children. I was raised to believe that children always come before any man. I was always taught that you were less than a woman if you put a man first. Can you explain this?

➡ The word of God says that we are to leave all others and cleave to our spouses. The Lord wants us to have a healthy balance in everything we do. However, God's

Word never tells us to neglect our children. When we talk about the husband being first, that is not at the expense of the children. Rather it is for the benefit of the children. In a healthy marriage, spouses must put priority on spending time with one another. This will give their children the script for how to conduct themselves in their future marriages. There is a serious problem when the parents are too wrapped up in the lives of their children and give little to no attention to the marriage. This is usually evidenced when couples experience the empty nest stage. There is a normal sense of loss.

Yet, some marriages are unable to stand because the marriage was out of balance with the children. Eventually the children will be grown and gone. Where will that leave those parents who have not prioritized their own relationships? Sadly many end up at the divorce courts.

9. My husband and I have been married for 2 years. We have a pretty good marriage. The only time we really have problems is when we visit his mother. She doesn't like the way I'm bringing up our daughter. In fact, she doesn't really like anything about me. I find myself under constant attack. I try to put up with her for my husband's sake. Whenever, he's not around, she says really nasty things to me. I love God. But my

flesh is definitely tried. I feel so beaten up by her. What should I do?

→ Many parents have a hard time letting go of their children when they get married. It seems your mother-in-law is having a hard time adjusting and she is taking out her frustration on you. You must let your husband know what is going on. Ask him to be aware of how she talks to you. He needs to be the one to confront her. She doesn't want to lose her son.
So she is more apt to listen to him than to you. She needs reassurance that she will always be an important part of your life. But at the same time, he must let her know that when she disrespects you, she disrespects him.

You are now one. So she cannot have the same place she had before you were married. Try to be understanding of the loss she feels. Pray that the Lord will minister to her.

Also pray for your husband. Sometimes, it is very difficult for a husband to confront his mother. The confrontation need not be combative. However, it is very necessary. He needs to make it clear to his extended family that he will tolerate nothing less than acceptance.

This will usually establish his manhood in the family. His mother has generally seen him as just her son. She needs to see him as a man with a family. He is still her son, but he is also an adult who is responsible to another family first.

10. We have been married 8 years. Our problem is that my husband is a jokester. He makes jokes at my expense. He will do anything to get a laugh. He talks about my weight, my cooking, my intelligence (or lack thereof), the way I dress. The list is exhaustive. It hurts my feelings so bad and it is destroying our relationship. Of course, he doesn't see it that way. He thinks that I over-react. And that I need to lighten up. He says laughter is his ministry. Please tell me what to do?

➡ Your husband needs to be sensitive to you. His ministry can NEVER be at the expense of his family.

He needs to recognize the damage that he is doing to you. The Bible says that life and death are in the power of the tongue. His put-downs are releasing death into your marriage. Respect is important in a marriage.

Your husband needs to discontinue his behavior just out of respect for you. When he starts with his putdowns, walk out of the room. Remove yourself from the situation. Do this every time. If this doesn't stop him, seek marriage counseling.

Recommitment Certificate

I, _____ and I, _____

do recommit our love and fidelity to the Lord, first, and then toward one another. We promise to love, honor, and respect each other. We will put each other first according to God's holy ordinance. We promise to forgive each other quickly, the same way, we want to receive it. We will stand for our marriage, no matter what obstacles we face. We will not give up, but persevere. We pledge to continually pray for each other.

We promise to love and support one another. And do everything in our power to keep this marriage alive and flourishing. We recognize that marriage is God's design. We will work together to glorify Him in this union. We believe in our union as marriage for a lifetime.

We will honor the Lord with this special gift that He has given to us. We will lovingly submit to the His word regarding our marriage.

So today, we renew the vows that we took on our wedding day. And we recommit our relationship to the Lord in the sight of God and the witnesses present this 13th day of February, 2010.

Husband's signature _____

Wife's signature _____

About the Authors

Apostle Oscar & Prophetess Crystal Jones

have been celebrating their covenant love for over 28 years. Their passion for one another has yielded a great harvest. They have 5 children and one daughter in law: Jake & Keila, Kyria, Charity, LaTina, and Christopher. They also delight in their 4 precious grandchildren: Kristin D'Ashley, Arielle Joy, Jaiman Jakehi, and Elijah Christopher.

Oscar & Crystal are both teachers by trade. They have taught in both the private and public sectors. Oscar has taught for both Detroit Public Schools and Oakland Unified Schools. He has recently left teaching after 27 years to pursue fulltime ministry. Prophetess Crystal is a licensed and practicing realtor for Century 21 Professional realtors.

Pastors Oscar & Crystal have an apostolic and prophetic mandate. They oversee **Greater Works Family Ministries** in Detroit, MI**, Marriage For A Lifetime Ministries** in Detroit, MI. They are founders of **Agape International Association of Churches and Parachurches** and **Alive Christian Fellowship** of Oakland, California.

They are serious about kingdom building. The couple has hosted a weekly call-in radio broadcast called **Grounds For Marriage** where they discussed issues relevant to marriage and the family. They have also been featured guests on several radio and television broadcasts.

The couple has co-authored a book entitled, **"When The Vow Breaks"** which is now in its second printing. They aspire to leave a legacy of hope and healing to marriages all over the world.

These long-time honeymooners continue to have a passion for marriage ministry. They have a unique team ministry where they speak together as one voice. They are in demand as conference speakers. To book them at your conference you may write to:

Marriage For A Lifetime Ministries
P.O. Box 24906
Oakland, CA 94623
Email: jones@marriage4alifetime.org
Website: www.marriage4alifetime.org

Also on Facebook and Twitter

Notes:

_____
_____
_____
_____
_____
_____
_____
_____
_____
_____
_____
_____
_____
_____
_____
_____
_____
_____
_____
_____
_____
_____
_____
_____
_____
_____
_____

Notes:

15382836R00076

Made in the USA
Charleston, SC
31 October 2012